This letters to my baby in heaven

IS DEDICATED TO:

_____

DEDICATION

This book is dedicated to all the hurting hearts out there.

You are my inspiration in producing books especially when the words will not come.

How to Use this Letters To My Baby In Heaven Diary:

The purpose of this Letters to My Baby is to keep all your various heart feels and thoughts organized in one easy to find spot.

Here are some simple guidelines to follow so you can make the most of using this book:

1. The first "Dear Baby I Found Out About You" section is for you to write out the date you found out about your baby on the way, how you felt. So you can go back there to be reminded of your journey.

2. Most ideas are inspired by something we have seen. Use the "How You Left Us" section to write down all the things you remember about that day.

3. The "My First Impressions of You Were" section is for you to write out all the things you loved about your baby, first thoughts, your journey.

4. And even more pages with the "What I Wanted You To Know About Me" section is great for writing out what you wanted your baby to know about you as a mom, a dad, grandparent or any member of the family.

5. The "When I Meet You In Heaven We Will" section is for you to keep a visual reminder of each dream you have for things and plans you have when you are reunited in heaven.

6. The "Your First Home Was Like This" section is for you to describe to your baby what his/her home was like, describe the fun places to play, toys to play with, any siblings looking forward to the baby's arrival so your heart feels understood.

7. The "My Favorite Pregnant Story Of You Is" section is for you to write all favorite stories to baby about things that happened while pregnant, favorite cravings, any heart feels especially helpful for remembering later on.

8. The "Things We Did While You Were Just A Bump" section is for you to write out keepsake memories of the fun-times, events, books read as your baby bump grew your story, your journey so your heart feels listened to.

9. Use this "On Your Birthday I Will Honor You By" section as the place to lay out your plan for honoring the baby on this day, a space for notes, how you envision the celebration so that your heart will feel understood... And much more!

Whether you're a first time parent or have been at it for a while, you will want to write down all your heart feels in this notebook to look back on and always remember all the things you want to say to your baby in heaven.

Enjoy!

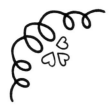
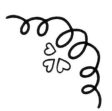

LETTERS TO MY *Baby* IN HEAVEN

Dear baby, the day i found out about you...

How you left us...

My first impressions of you were...

What I wanted you to know about me was...

When I meet you in heaven we will...

Your first home was like this...

My favorite pregnant story of you is...

Things we did while you were just a bump...

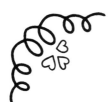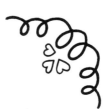

LETTERS TO MY *Baby* IN HEAVEN

We chose to name you...

My bucket list for you was...

The first thing we will do together when I see you in heaven is...

I know that God needed another angel...

And I imagine right now your job in heaven is...

I want to share this bible verse with you...

Some lessons I learned from just knowing you are...

On your birthday I will honor you by...

My faith has changed in these ways...

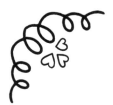 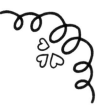

LETTERS TO MY *Baby* IN HEAVEN

I just wanted to tell you...

My list of words that describe you are...

When I think of you and the fun times we were gonna have, I imagine it like this...

When I get sad cause I miss you, I do this....

What I wish others knew about you is...

Notes

LETTERS TO MY *Baby* IN HEAVEN

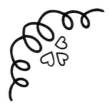 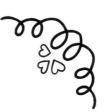

LETTERS TO MY *Baby* IN HEAVEN

Dear baby, the day i found out about you...

How you left us...

My first impressions of you were...

What I wanted you to know about me was...

When I meet you in heaven we will...

Your first home was like this...

My favorite pregnant story of you is...

Things we did while you were just a bump...

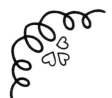
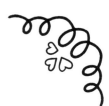

LETTERS TO MY *Baby* IN HEAVEN

We chose to name you...

My bucket list for you was...

The first thing we will do together when I see you in heaven is...

I know that God needed another angel...

And I imagine right now your job in heaven is...

I want to share this bible verse with you...

Some lessons I learned from just knowing you are...

On your birthday I will honor you by...

My faith has changed in these ways...

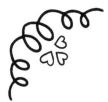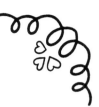

LETTERS TO MY *Baby* IN HEAVEN

I just wanted to tell you...

My list of words that describe you are...

When I think of you and the fun times we were gonna have, I imagine it like this...

When I get sad cause I miss you, I do this....

What I wish others knew about you is...

Notes

LETTERS TO MY *Baby* IN HEAVEN

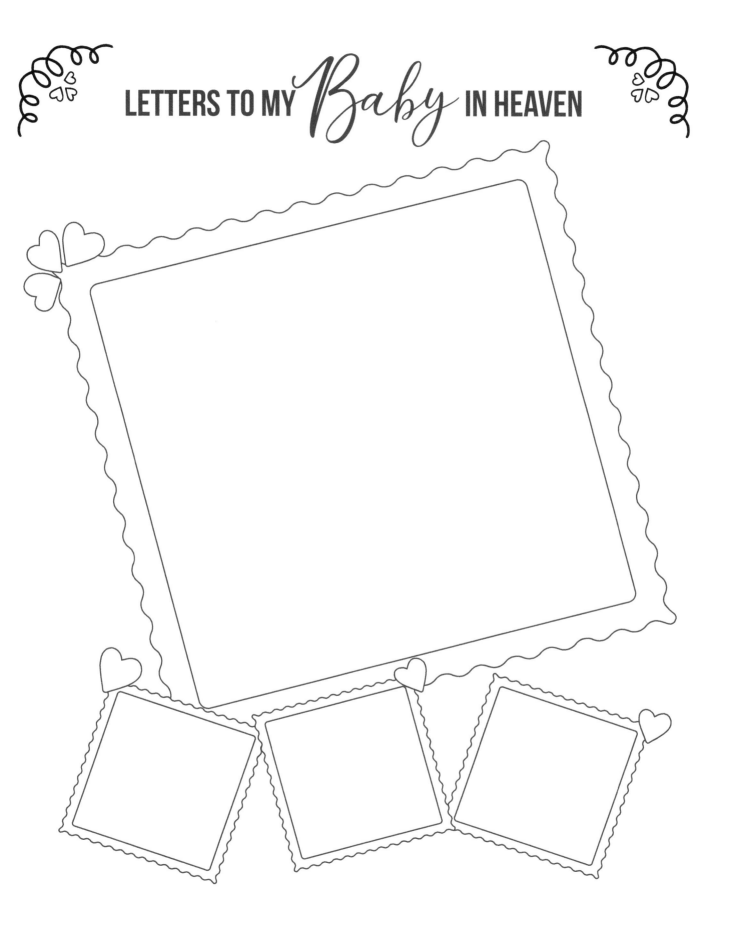

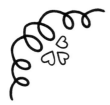
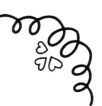

LETTERS TO MY *Baby* IN HEAVEN

Dear baby, the day i found out about you...

How you left us...

My first impressions of you were...

What I wanted you to know about me was...

When I meet you in heaven we will...

Your first home was like this...

My favorite pregnant story of you is...

Things we did while you were just a bump...

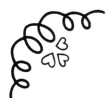
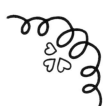

LETTERS TO MY *Baby* IN HEAVEN

We chose to name you...

My bucket list for you was...

The first thing we will do together when I see you in heaven is...

I know that God needed another angel...

And I imagine right now your job in heaven is...

I want to share this bible verse with you...

Some lessons I learned from just knowing you are...

On your birthday I will honor you by...

My faith has changed in these ways...

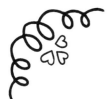 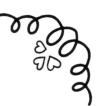

LETTERS TO MY *Baby* IN HEAVEN

I just wanted to tell you...

My list of words that describe you are...

When I think of you and the fun times we were gonna have, I imagine it like this...

When I get sad cause I miss you, I do this....

What I wish others knew about you is...

Notes

LETTERS TO MY *Baby* IN HEAVEN

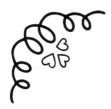 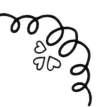

LETTERS TO MY *Baby* IN HEAVEN

Dear baby, the day i found out about you...

How you left us...

My first impressions of you were...

What I wanted you to know about me was...

When I meet you in heaven we will...

Your first home was like this...

My favorite pregnant story of you is...

Things we did while you were just a bump...

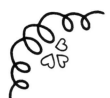
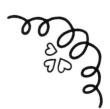

LETTERS TO MY *Baby* IN HEAVEN

We chose to name you...

My bucket list for you was...

The first thing we will do together when I see you in heaven is...

I know that God needed another angel...

And I imagine right now your job in heaven is...

I want to share this bible verse with you...

Some lessons I learned from just knowing you are...

On your birthday I will honor you by...

My faith has changed in these ways...

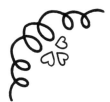 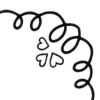

LETTERS TO MY *Baby* IN HEAVEN

I just wanted to tell you...

My list of words that describe you are...

When I think of you and the fun times we were gonna have, I imagine it like this...

When I get sad cause I miss you, I do this....

What I wish others knew about you is...

Notes

LETTERS TO MY *Baby* IN HEAVEN

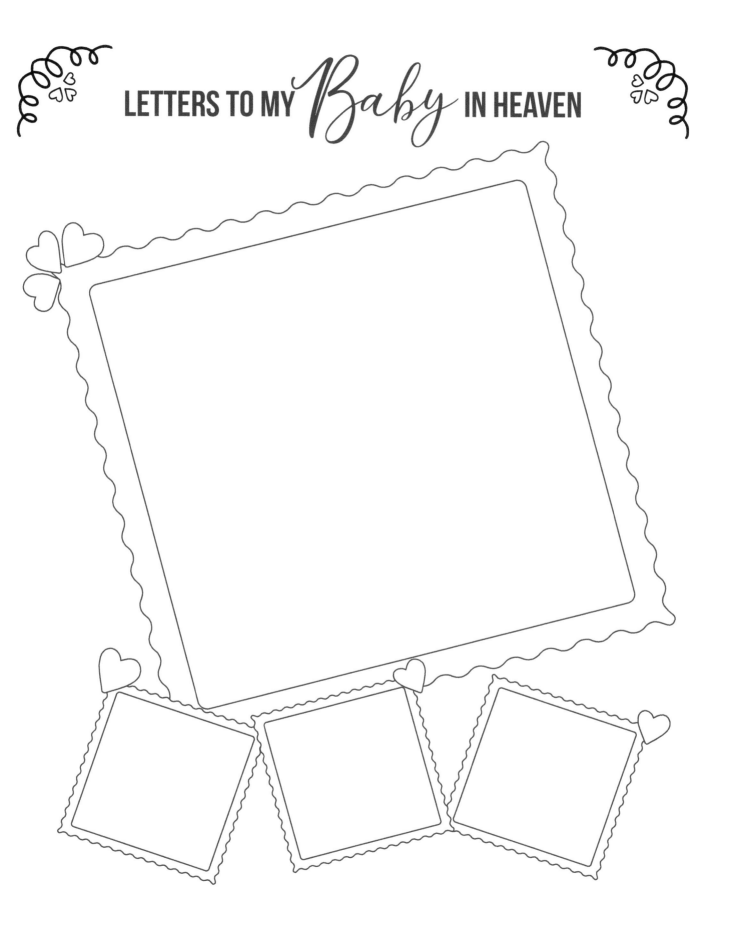

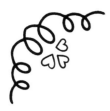 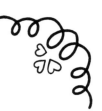

LETTERS TO MY *Baby* IN HEAVEN

Dear baby, the day i found out about you...

How you left us...

My first impressions of you were...

What I wanted you to know about me was...

When I meet you in heaven we will...

Your first home was like this...

My favorite pregnant story of you is...

Things we did while you were just a bump...

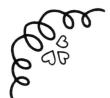 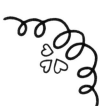

LETTERS TO MY *Baby* IN HEAVEN

We chose to name you...

My bucket list for you was...

The first thing we will do together when I see you in heaven is...

I know that God needed another angel...

And I imagine right now your job in heaven is...

I want to share this bible verse with you...

Some lessons I learned from just knowing you are...

On your birthday I will honor you by...

My faith has changed in these ways...

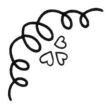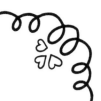

LETTERS TO MY *Baby* IN HEAVEN

I just wanted to tell you...

My list of words that describe you are...

When I think of you and the fun times we were gonna have, I imagine it like this...

When I get sad cause I miss you, I do this....

What I wish others knew about you is...

Notes

LETTERS TO MY *Baby* IN HEAVEN

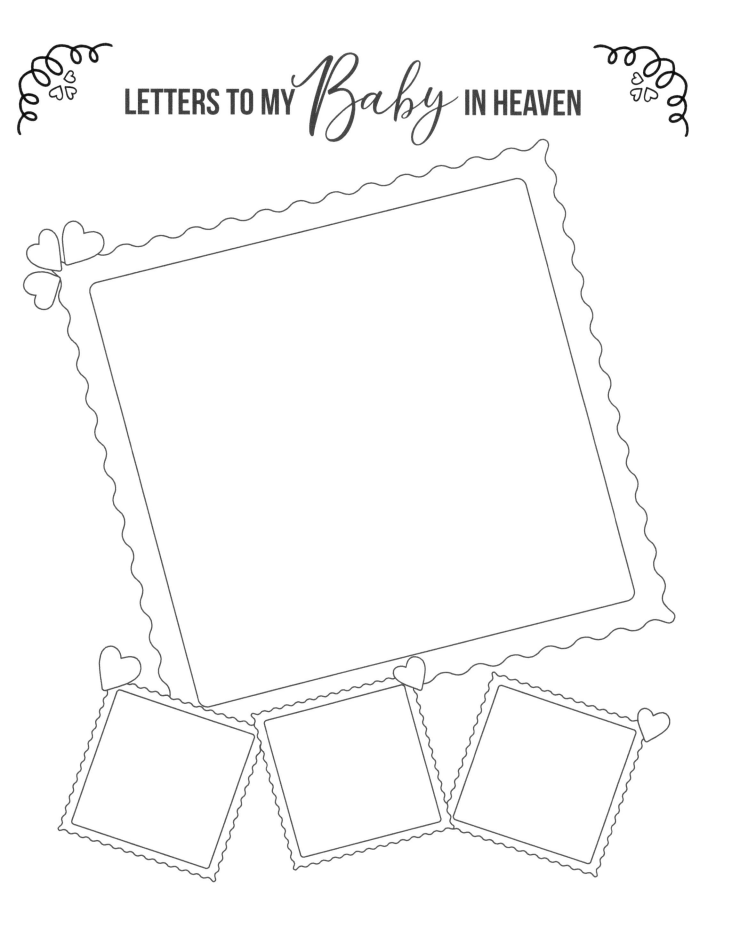

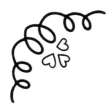
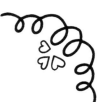

LETTERS TO MY *Baby* IN HEAVEN

Dear baby, the day i found out about you...

How you left us...

My first impressions of you were...

What I wanted you to know about me was...

When I meet you in heaven we will...

Your first home was like this...

My favorite pregnant story of you is...

Things we did while you were just a bump...

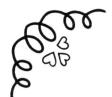 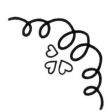

LETTERS TO MY *Baby* IN HEAVEN

We chose to name you...

My bucket list for you was...

The first thing we will do together when I see you in heaven is...

I know that God needed another angel...

And I imagine right now your job in heaven is...

I want to share this bible verse with you...

Some lessons I learned from just knowing you are...

On your birthday I will honor you by...

My faith has changed in these ways...

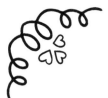 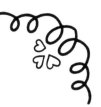

LETTERS TO MY *Baby* IN HEAVEN

I just wanted to tell you...

My list of words that describe you are...

When I think of you and the fun times we were gonna have, I imagine it like this...

When I get sad cause I miss you, I do this....

What I wish others knew about you is...

Notes

LETTERS TO MY *Baby* IN HEAVEN

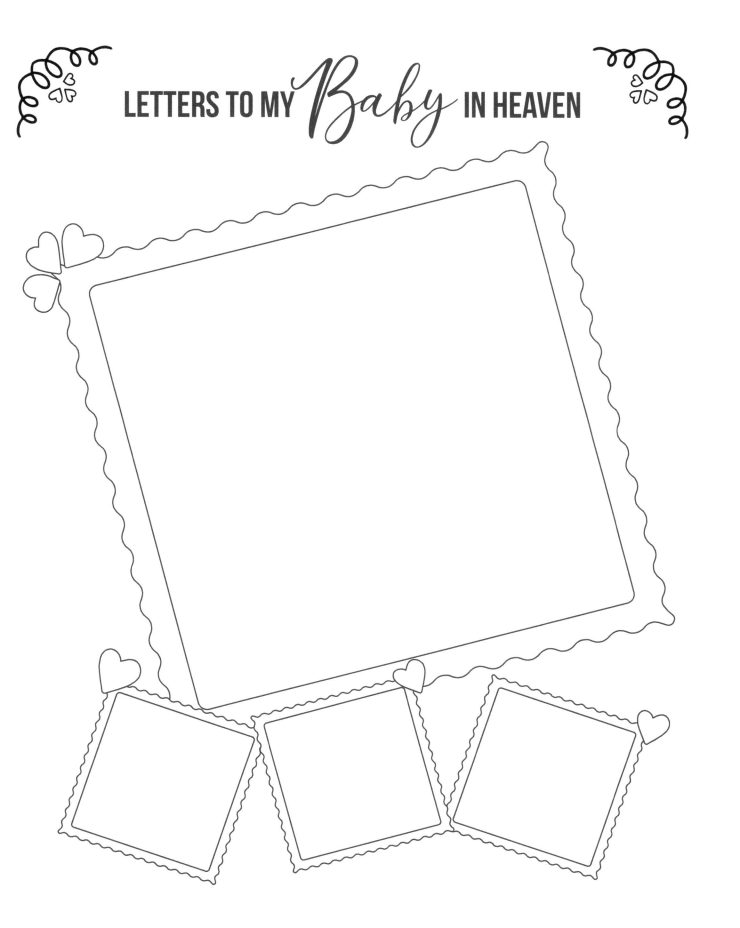

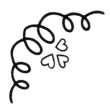
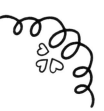

LETTERS TO MY *Baby* IN HEAVEN

Dear baby, the day i found out about you...

How you left us...

My first impressions of you were...

What I wanted you to know about me was...

When I meet you in heaven we will...

Your first home was like this...

My favorite pregnant story of you is...

Things we did while you were just a bump...

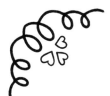 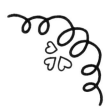

LETTERS TO MY *Baby* IN HEAVEN

We chose to name you...

My bucket list for you was...

The first thing we will do together when I see you in heaven is...

I know that God needed another angel...

And I imagine right now your job in heaven is...

I want to share this bible verse with you...

Some lessons I learned from just knowing you are...

On your birthday I will honor you by...

My faith has changed in these ways...

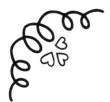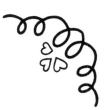

LETTERS TO MY *Baby* IN HEAVEN

I just wanted to tell you...

My list of words that describe you are...

When I think of you and the fun times we were gonna have, I imagine it like this...

When I get sad cause I miss you, I do this....

What I wish others knew about you is...

Notes

LETTERS TO MY *Baby* IN HEAVEN

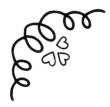
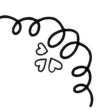

LETTERS TO MY *Baby* IN HEAVEN

Dear baby, the day i found out about you...

How you left us...

My first impressions of you were...

What I wanted you to know about me was...

When I meet you in heaven we will...

Your first home was like this...

My favorite pregnant story of you is...

Things we did while you were just a bump...

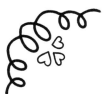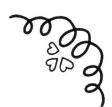

LETTERS TO MY *Baby* IN HEAVEN

We chose to name you...

My bucket list for you was...

The first thing we will do together when I see you in heaven is...

I know that God needed another angel...

And I imagine right now your job in heaven is...

I want to share this bible verse with you...

Some lessons I learned from just knowing you are...

On your birthday I will honor you by...

My faith has changed in these ways...

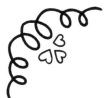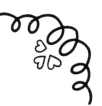

LETTERS TO MY *Baby* IN HEAVEN

I just wanted to tell you...

My list of words that describe you are...

When I think of you and the fun times we were gonna have, I imagine it like this...

When I get sad cause I miss you, I do this....

What I wish others knew about you is...

Notes

LETTERS TO MY *Baby* IN HEAVEN

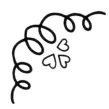 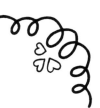

LETTERS TO MY *Baby* IN HEAVEN

Dear baby, the day i found out about you...

How you left us...

My first impressions of you were...

What I wanted you to know about me was...

When I meet you in heaven we will...

Your first home was like this...

My favorite pregnant story of you is...

Things we did while you were just a bump...

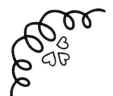
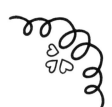

LETTERS TO MY *Baby* IN HEAVEN

We chose to name you...

My bucket list for you was...

The first thing we will do together when I see you in heaven is...

I know that God needed another angel...

And I imagine right now your job in heaven is...

I want to share this bible verse with you...

Some lessons I learned from just knowing you are...

On your birthday I will honor you by...

My faith has changed in these ways...

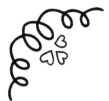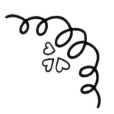

LETTERS TO MY *Baby* IN HEAVEN

I just wanted to tell you...

My list of words that describe you are...

When I think of you and the fun times we were gonna have, I imagine it like this...

When I get sad cause I miss you, I do this....

What I wish others knew about you is...

Notes

LETTERS TO MY *Baby* IN HEAVEN

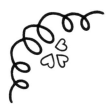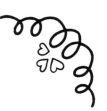

LETTERS TO MY *Baby* IN HEAVEN

Dear baby, the day i found out about you...

How you left us...

My first impressions of you were...

What I wanted you to know about me was...

When I meet you in heaven we will...

Your first home was like this...

My favorite pregnant story of you is...

Things we did while you were just a bump...

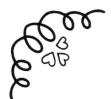 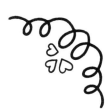

LETTERS TO MY *Baby* IN HEAVEN

We chose to name you...

My bucket list for you was...

The first thing we will do together when I see you in heaven is...

I know that God needed another angel...

And I imagine right now your job in heaven is...

I want to share this bible verse with you...

Some lessons I learned from just knowing you are...

On your birthday I will honor you by...

My faith has changed in these ways...

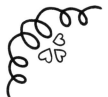 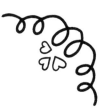

LETTERS TO MY *Baby* IN HEAVEN

I just wanted to tell you...

My list of words that describe you are...

When I think of you and the fun times we were gonna have, I imagine it like this...

When I get sad cause I miss you, I do this....

What I wish others knew about you is...

Notes

LETTERS TO MY *Baby* IN HEAVEN

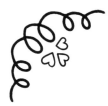
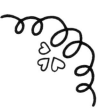

LETTERS TO MY *Baby* IN HEAVEN

Dear baby, the day i found out about you...

How you left us...

My first impressions of you were...

What I wanted you to know about me was...

When I meet you in heaven we will...

Your first home was like this...

My favorite pregnant story of you is...

Things we did while you were just a bump...

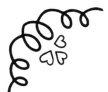
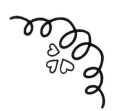

LETTERS TO MY *Baby* IN HEAVEN

We chose to name you...

My bucket list for you was...

The first thing we will do together when I see you in heaven is...

I know that God needed another angel...

And I imagine right now your job in heaven is...

I want to share this bible verse with you...

Some lessons I learned from just knowing you are...

On your birthday I will honor you by...

My faith has changed in these ways...

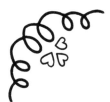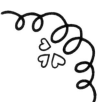

LETTERS TO MY *Baby* IN HEAVEN

I just wanted to tell you...

My list of words that describe you are...

When I think of you and the fun times we were gonna have, I imagine it like this...

When I get sad cause I miss you, I do this....

What I wish others knew about you is...

Notes

LETTERS TO MY *Baby* IN HEAVEN

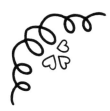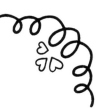

LETTERS TO MY *Baby* IN HEAVEN

Dear baby, the day i found out about you...

How you left us...

My first impressions of you were...

What I wanted you to know about me was...

When I meet you in heaven we will...

Your first home was like this...

My favorite pregnant story of you is...

Things we did while you were just a bump...

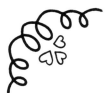 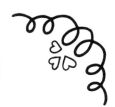

LETTERS TO MY *Baby* IN HEAVEN

We chose to name you...

My bucket list for you was...

The first thing we will do together when I see you in heaven is...

I know that God needed another angel...

And I imagine right now your job in heaven is...

I want to share this bible verse with you...

Some lessons I learned from just knowing you are...

On your birthday I will honor you by...

My faith has changed in these ways...

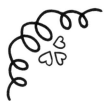 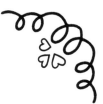

LETTERS TO MY *Baby* IN HEAVEN

I just wanted to tell you...

My list of words that describe you are...

When I think of you and the fun times we were gonna have, I imagine it like this...

When I get sad cause I miss you, I do this....

What I wish others knew about you is...

Notes

LETTERS TO MY *Baby* IN HEAVEN

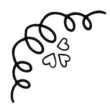
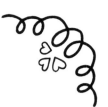

LETTERS TO MY *Baby* IN HEAVEN

Dear baby, the day i found out about you...

How you left us...

My first impressions of you were...

What I wanted you to know about me was...

When I meet you in heaven we will...

Your first home was like this...

My favorite pregnant story of you is...

Things we did while you were just a bump...

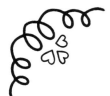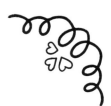

LETTERS TO MY *Baby* IN HEAVEN

We chose to name you...

My bucket list for you was...

The first thing we will do together when I see you in heaven is...

I know that God needed another angel...

And I imagine right now your job in heaven is...

I want to share this bible verse with you...

Some lessons I learned from just knowing you are...

On your birthday I will honor you by...

My faith has changed in these ways...

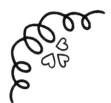 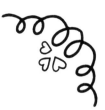

LETTERS TO MY *Baby* IN HEAVEN

I just wanted to tell you...

My list of words that describe you are...

When I think of you and the fun times we were gonna have, I imagine it like this...

When I get sad cause I miss you, I do this....

What I wish others knew about you is...

Notes

LETTERS TO MY *Baby* IN HEAVEN

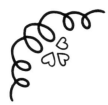
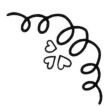

LETTERS TO MY *Baby* IN HEAVEN

Dear baby, the day i found out about you...

How you left us...

My first impressions of you were...

What I wanted you to know about me was...

When I meet you in heaven we will...

Your first home was like this...

My favorite pregnant story of you is...

Things we did while you were just a bump...

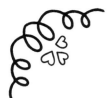
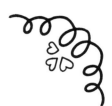

LETTERS TO MY *Baby* IN HEAVEN

We chose to name you...

My bucket list for you was...

The first thing we will do together when I see you in heaven is...

I know that God needed another angel...

And I imagine right now your job in heaven is...

I want to share this bible verse with you...

Some lessons I learned from just knowing you are...

On your birthday I will honor you by...

My faith has changed in these ways...

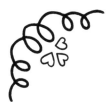 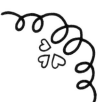

LETTERS TO MY *Baby* IN HEAVEN

I just wanted to tell you...

My list of words that describe you are...

When I think of you and the fun times we were gonna have, I imagine it like this...

When I get sad cause I miss you, I do this....

What I wish others knew about you is...

Notes

LETTERS TO MY *Baby* IN HEAVEN

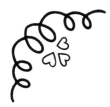 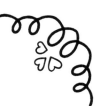

LETTERS TO MY *Baby* IN HEAVEN

Dear baby, the day i found out about you...

How you left us...

My first impressions of you were...

What I wanted you to know about me was...

When I meet you in heaven we will...

Your first home was like this...

My favorite pregnant story of you is...

Things we did while you were just a bump...

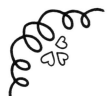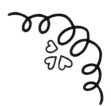

LETTERS TO MY *Baby* IN HEAVEN

We chose to name you...

My bucket list for you was...

The first thing we will do together when I see you in heaven is...

I know that God needed another angel...

And I imagine right now your job in heaven is...

I want to share this bible verse with you...

Some lessons I learned from just knowing you are...

On your birthday I will honor you by...

My faith has changed in these ways...

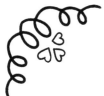 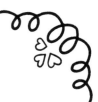

LETTERS TO MY *Baby* IN HEAVEN

I just wanted to tell you...

My list of words that describe you are...

When I think of you and the fun times we were gonna have, I imagine it like this...

When I get sad cause I miss you, I do this....

What I wish others knew about you is...

Notes

LETTERS TO MY *Baby* IN HEAVEN

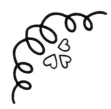
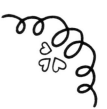

LETTERS TO MY *Baby* IN HEAVEN

Dear baby, the day i found out about you...

How you left us...

My first impressions of you were...

What I wanted you to know about me was...

When I meet you in heaven we will...

Your first home was like this...

My favorite pregnant story of you is...

Things we did while you were just a bump...

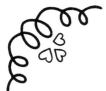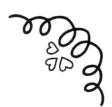

LETTERS TO MY *Baby* IN HEAVEN

We chose to name you...

My bucket list for you was...

The first thing we will do together when I see you in heaven is...

I know that God needed another angel...

And I imagine right now your job in heaven is...

I want to share this bible verse with you...

Some lessons I learned from just knowing you are...

On your birthday I will honor you by...

My faith has changed in these ways...

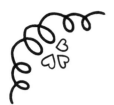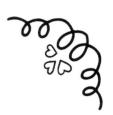

LETTERS TO MY *Baby* IN HEAVEN

I just wanted to tell you...

My list of words that describe you are...

When I think of you and the fun times we were gonna have, I imagine it like this...

When I get sad cause I miss you, I do this....

What I wish others knew about you is...

Notes

LETTERS TO MY *Baby* IN HEAVEN

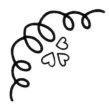 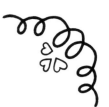

LETTERS TO MY *Baby* IN HEAVEN

Dear baby, the day i found out about you...

How you left us...

My first impressions of you were...

What I wanted you to know about me was...

When I meet you in heaven we will...

Your first home was like this...

My favorite pregnant story of you is...

Things we did while you were just a bump...

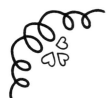
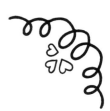

LETTERS TO MY *Baby* IN HEAVEN

We chose to name you...

My bucket list for you was...

The first thing we will do together when I see you in heaven is...

I know that God needed another angel...

And I imagine right now your job in heaven is...

I want to share this bible verse with you...

Some lessons I learned from just knowing you are...

On your birthday I will honor you by...

My faith has changed in these ways...

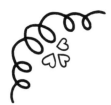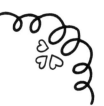

LETTERS TO MY *Baby* IN HEAVEN

I just wanted to tell you...

My list of words that describe you are...

When I think of you and the fun times we were gonna have, I imagine it like this...

When I get sad cause I miss you, I do this....

What I wish others knew about you is...

Notes

LETTERS TO MY *Baby* IN HEAVEN

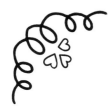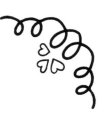

LETTERS TO MY *Baby* IN HEAVEN

Dear baby, the day i found out about you...

How you left us...

My first impressions of you were...

What I wanted you to know about me was...

When I meet you in heaven we will...

Your first home was like this...

My favorite pregnant story of you is...

Things we did while you were just a bump...

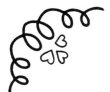
LETTERS TO MY *Baby* IN HEAVEN
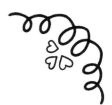

We chose to name you...

My bucket list for you was...

The first thing we will do together when I see you in heaven is...

I know that God needed another angel...

And I imagine right now your job in heaven is...

I want to share this bible verse with you...

Some lessons I learned from just knowing you are...

On your birthday I will honor you by...

My faith has changed in these ways...

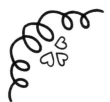 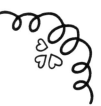

LETTERS TO MY *Baby* IN HEAVEN

I just wanted to tell you...

My list of words that describe you are...

When I think of you and the fun times we were gonna have, I imagine it like this...

When I get sad cause I miss you, I do this....

What I wish others knew about you is...

Notes

LETTERS TO MY *Baby* IN HEAVEN

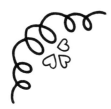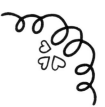

LETTERS TO MY *Baby* IN HEAVEN

Dear baby, the day i found out about you...

How you left us...

My first impressions of you were...

What I wanted you to know about me was...

When I meet you in heaven we will...

Your first home was like this...

My favorite pregnant story of you is...

Things we did while you were just a bump...

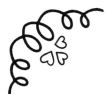
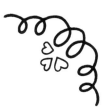

LETTERS TO MY *Baby* IN HEAVEN

We chose to name you...

My bucket list for you was...

The first thing we will do together when I see you in heaven is...

I know that God needed another angel...

And I imagine right now your job in heaven is...

I want to share this bible verse with you...

Some lessons I learned from just knowing you are...

On your birthday I will honor you by...

My faith has changed in these ways...

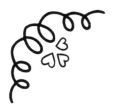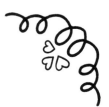

LETTERS TO MY *Baby* IN HEAVEN

I just wanted to tell you...

My list of words that describe you are...

When I think of you and the fun times we were gonna have, I imagine it like this...

When I get sad cause I miss you, I do this....

What I wish others knew about you is...

Notes

LETTERS TO MY *Baby* IN HEAVEN

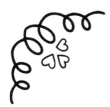
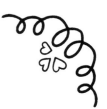

LETTERS TO MY *Baby* IN HEAVEN

Dear baby, the day i found out about you...

How you left us...

My first impressions of you were...

What I wanted you to know about me was...

When I meet you in heaven we will...

Your first home was like this...

My favorite pregnant story of you is...

Things we did while you were just a bump...

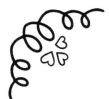 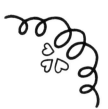

LETTERS TO MY *Baby* IN HEAVEN

We chose to name you...

My bucket list for you was...

The first thing we will do together when I see you in heaven is...

I know that God needed another angel...

And I imagine right now your job in heaven is...

I want to share this bible verse with you...

Some lessons I learned from just knowing you are...

On your birthday I will honor you by...

My faith has changed in these ways...

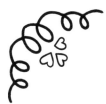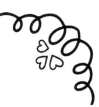

LETTERS TO MY *Baby* IN HEAVEN

I just wanted to tell you...

My list of words that describe you are...

When I think of you and the fun times we were gonna have, I imagine it like this...

When I get sad cause I miss you, I do this....

What I wish others knew about you is...

Notes

LETTERS TO MY *Baby* IN HEAVEN

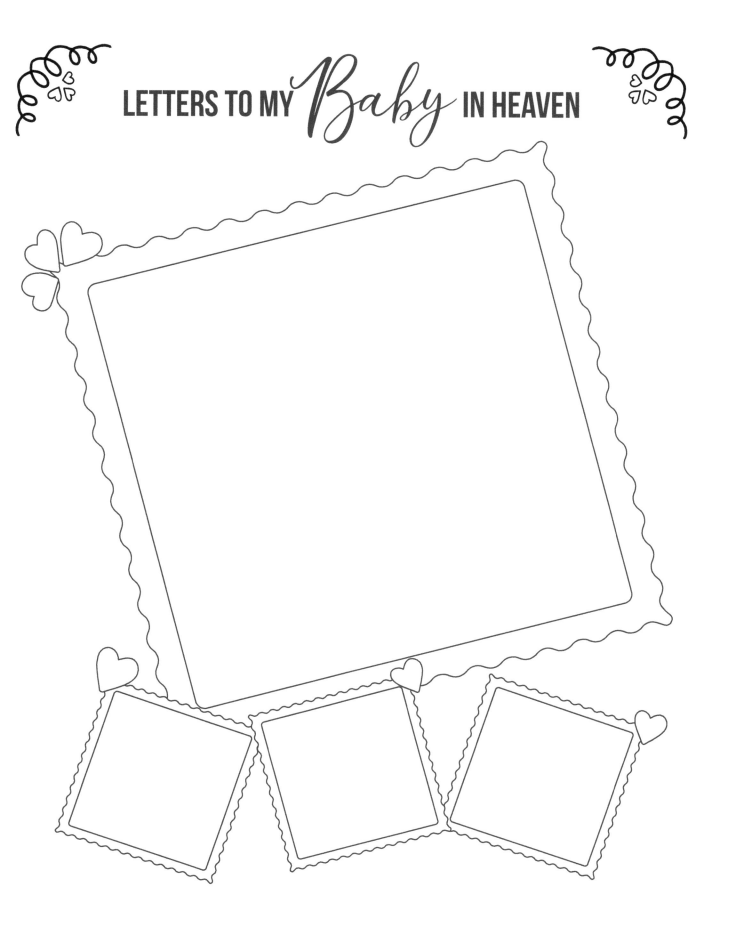

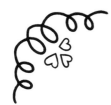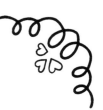

LETTERS TO MY *Baby* IN HEAVEN

Dear baby, the day i found out about you...

How you left us...

My first impressions of you were...

What I wanted you to know about me was...

When I meet you in heaven we will...

Your first home was like this...

My favorite pregnant story of you is...

Things we did while you were just a bump...

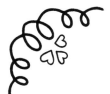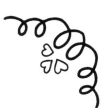

LETTERS TO MY *Baby* IN HEAVEN

We chose to name you...

My bucket list for you was...

The first thing we will do together when I see you in heaven is...

I know that God needed another angel...

And I imagine right now your job in heaven is...

I want to share this bible verse with you...

Some lessons I learned from just knowing you are...

On your birthday I will honor you by...

My faith has changed in these ways...

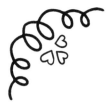
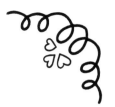

LETTERS TO MY *Baby* IN HEAVEN

I just wanted to tell you...

My list of words that describe you are...

When I think of you and the fun times we were gonna have, I imagine it like this...

When I get sad cause I miss you, I do this....

What I wish others knew about you is...

Notes

LETTERS TO MY *Baby* IN HEAVEN

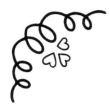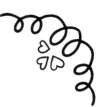

LETTERS TO MY *Baby* IN HEAVEN

Dear baby, the day i found out about you...

How you left us...

My first impressions of you were...

What I wanted you to know about me was...

When I meet you in heaven we will...

Your first home was like this...

My favorite pregnant story of you is...

Things we did while you were just a bump...

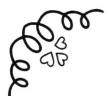
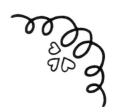

LETTERS TO MY *Baby* IN HEAVEN

We chose to name you...

My bucket list for you was...

The first thing we will do together when I see you in heaven is...

I know that God needed another angel...

And I imagine right now your job in heaven is...

I want to share this bible verse with you...

Some lessons I learned from just knowing you are...

On your birthday I will honor you by...

My faith has changed in these ways...

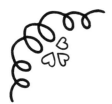 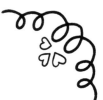

LETTERS TO MY *Baby* IN HEAVEN

I just wanted to tell you...

My list of words that describe you are...

When I think of you and the fun times we were gonna have, I imagine it like this...

When I get sad cause I miss you, I do this....

What I wish others knew about you is...

Notes

LETTERS TO MY *Baby* IN HEAVEN

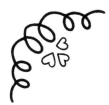
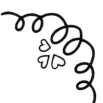

LETTERS TO MY *Baby* IN HEAVEN

Dear baby, the day i found out about you...

How you left us...

My first impressions of you were...

What I wanted you to know about me was...

When I meet you in heaven we will...

Your first home was like this...

My favorite pregnant story of you is...

Things we did while you were just a bump...

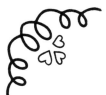 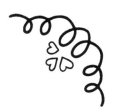

LETTERS TO MY *Baby* IN HEAVEN

We chose to name you...

My bucket list for you was...

The first thing we will do together when I see you in heaven is...

I know that God needed another angel...

And I imagine right now your job in heaven is...

I want to share this bible verse with you...

Some lessons I learned from just knowing you are...

On your birthday I will honor you by...

My faith has changed in these ways...

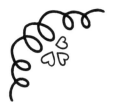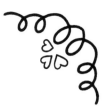

LETTERS TO MY *Baby* IN HEAVEN

I just wanted to tell you...

My list of words that describe you are...

When I think of you and the fun times we were gonna have, I imagine it like this...

When I get sad cause I miss you, I do this....

What I wish others knew about you is...

Notes

LETTERS TO MY *Baby* IN HEAVEN

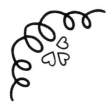
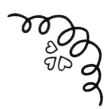

LETTERS TO MY *Baby* IN HEAVEN

Dear baby, the day i found out about you...

How you left us...

My first impressions of you were...

What I wanted you to know about me was...

When I meet you in heaven we will...

Your first home was like this...

My favorite pregnant story of you is...

Things we did while you were just a bump...

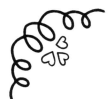 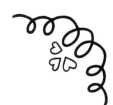

LETTERS TO MY *Baby* IN HEAVEN

We chose to name you...

My bucket list for you was...

The first thing we will do together when I see you in heaven is...

I know that God needed another angel...

And I imagine right now your job in heaven is...

I want to share this bible verse with you...

Some lessons I learned from just knowing you are...

On your birthday I will honor you by...

My faith has changed in these ways...

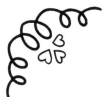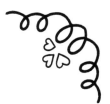

LETTERS TO MY *Baby* IN HEAVEN

I just wanted to tell you...

My list of words that describe you are...

When I think of you and the fun times we were gonna have, I imagine it like this...

When I get sad cause I miss you, I do this....

What I wish others knew about you is...

Notes

LETTERS TO MY *Baby* IN HEAVEN

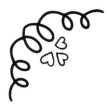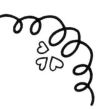

LETTERS TO MY *Baby* IN HEAVEN

Dear baby, the day i found out about you...

How you left us...

My first impressions of you were...

What I wanted you to know about me was...

When I meet you in heaven we will...

Your first home was like this...

My favorite pregnant story of you is...

Things we did while you were just a bump...

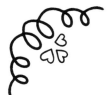 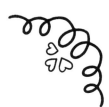

LETTERS TO MY *Baby* IN HEAVEN

We chose to name you...

My bucket list for you was...

The first thing we will do together when I see you in heaven is...

I know that God needed another angel...

And I imagine right now your job in heaven is...

I want to share this bible verse with you...

Some lessons I learned from just knowing you are...

On your birthday I will honor you by...

My faith has changed in these ways...

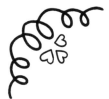 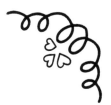

LETTERS TO MY *Baby* IN HEAVEN

I just wanted to tell you...

My list of words that describe you are...

When I think of you and the fun times we were gonna have, I imagine it like this...

When I get sad cause I miss you, I do this....

What I wish others knew about you is...

Notes

LETTERS TO MY *Baby* IN HEAVEN

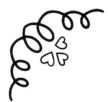
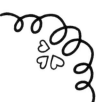

LETTERS TO MY *Baby* IN HEAVEN

Dear baby, the day i found out about you...

How you left us...

My first impressions of you were...

What I wanted you to know about me was...

When I meet you in heaven we will...

Your first home was like this...

My favorite pregnant story of you is...

Things we did while you were just a bump...

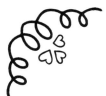
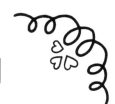

LETTERS TO MY *Baby* IN HEAVEN

We chose to name you...

My bucket list for you was...

The first thing we will do together when I see you in heaven is...

I know that God needed another angel...

And I imagine right now your job in heaven is...

I want to share this bible verse with you...

Some lessons I learned from just knowing you are...

On your birthday I will honor you by...

My faith has changed in these ways...

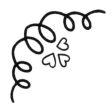 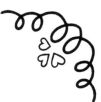

LETTERS TO MY *Baby* IN HEAVEN

I just wanted to tell you...

My list of words that describe you are...

When I think of you and the fun times we were gonna have, I imagine it like this...

When I get sad cause I miss you, I do this....

What I wish others knew about you is...

Notes

LETTERS TO MY *Baby* IN HEAVEN

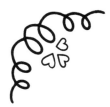 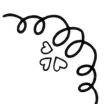

LETTERS TO MY *Baby* IN HEAVEN

Dear baby, the day i found out about you...

How you left us...

My first impressions of you were...

What I wanted you to know about me was...

When I meet you in heaven we will...

Your first home was like this...

My favorite pregnant story of you is...

Things we did while you were just a bump...

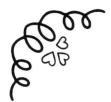 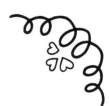

LETTERS TO MY *Baby* IN HEAVEN

We chose to name you...

My bucket list for you was...

The first thing we will do together when I see you in heaven is...

I know that God needed another angel...

And I imagine right now your job in heaven is...

I want to share this bible verse with you...

Some lessons I learned from just knowing you are...

On your birthday I will honor you by...

My faith has changed in these ways...

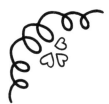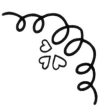

LETTERS TO MY *Baby* IN HEAVEN

I just wanted to tell you...

My list of words that describe you are...

When I think of you and the fun times we were gonna have, I imagine it like this...

When I get sad cause I miss you, I do this....

What I wish others knew about you is...

Notes

LETTERS TO MY *Baby* IN HEAVEN

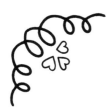 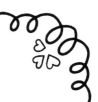

LETTERS TO MY *Baby* IN HEAVEN

Dear baby, the day i found out about you...

How you left us...

My first impressions of you were...

What I wanted you to know about me was...

When I meet you in heaven we will...

Your first home was like this...

My favorite pregnant story of you is...

Things we did while you were just a bump...

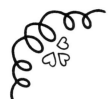
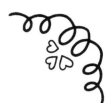

LETTERS TO MY *Baby* IN HEAVEN

We chose to name you...

My bucket list for you was...

The first thing we will do together when I see you in heaven is...

I know that God needed another angel...

And I imagine right now your job in heaven is...

I want to share this bible verse with you...

Some lessons I learned from just knowing you are...

On your birthday I will honor you by...

My faith has changed in these ways...

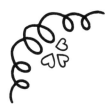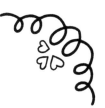

LETTERS TO MY *Baby* IN HEAVEN

I just wanted to tell you...

My list of words that describe you are...

When I think of you and the fun times we were gonna have, I imagine it like this...

When I get sad cause I miss you, I do this....

What I wish others knew about you is...

Notes

LETTERS TO MY *Baby* IN HEAVEN

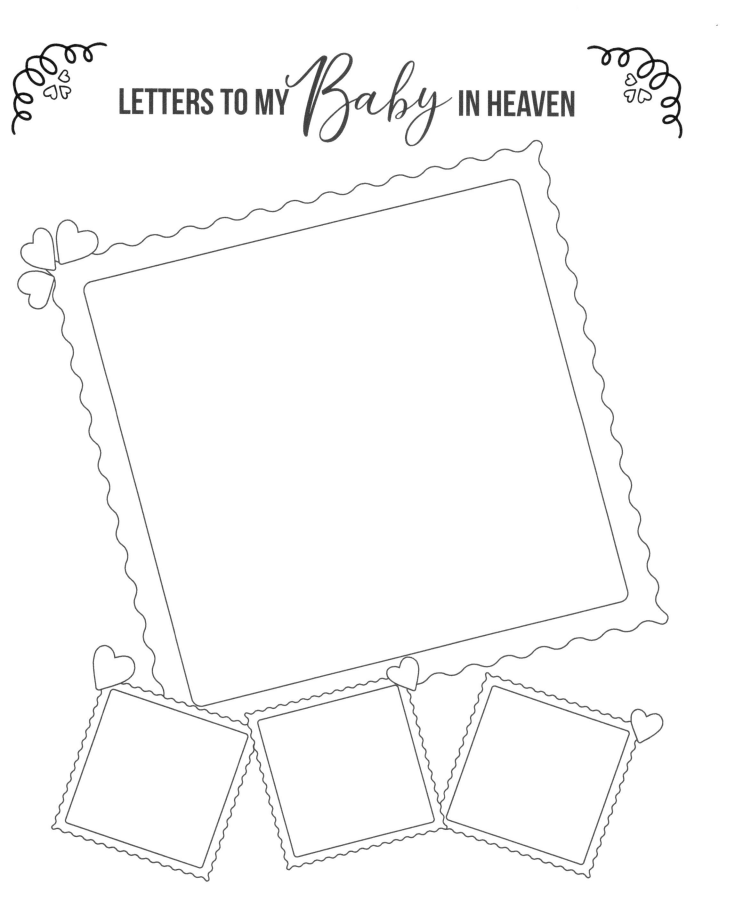

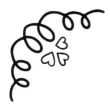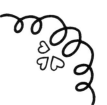

LETTERS TO MY *Baby* IN HEAVEN

Dear baby, the day i found out about you...

How you left us...

My first impressions of you were...

What I wanted you to know about me was...

When I meet you in heaven we will...

Your first home was like this...

My favorite pregnant story of you is...

Things we did while you were just a bump...

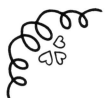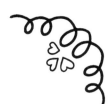

LETTERS TO MY *Baby* IN HEAVEN

We chose to name you...

My bucket list for you was...

The first thing we will do together when I see you in heaven is...

I know that God needed another angel...

And I imagine right now your job in heaven is...

I want to share this bible verse with you...

Some lessons I learned from just knowing you are...

On your birthday I will honor you by...

My faith has changed in these ways...

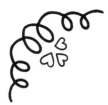
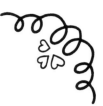

LETTERS TO MY *Baby* IN HEAVEN

I just wanted to tell you...

My list of words that describe you are...

When I think of you and the fun times we were gonna have, I imagine it like this...

When I get sad cause I miss you, I do this....

What I wish others knew about you is...

Notes

LETTERS TO MY *Baby* IN HEAVEN

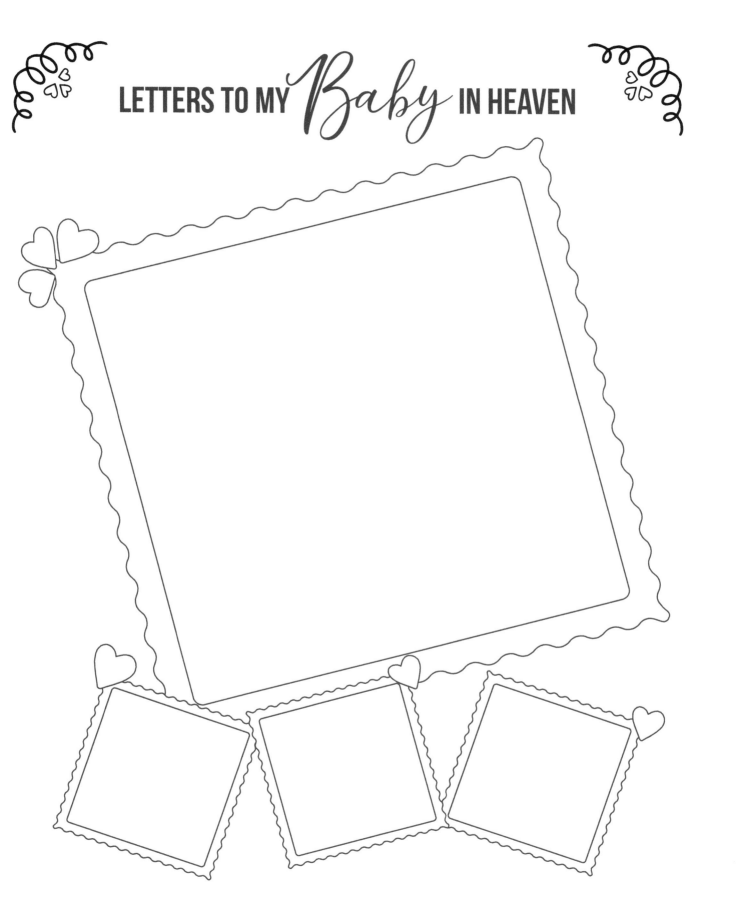

LETTERS TO MY *Baby* IN HEAVEN

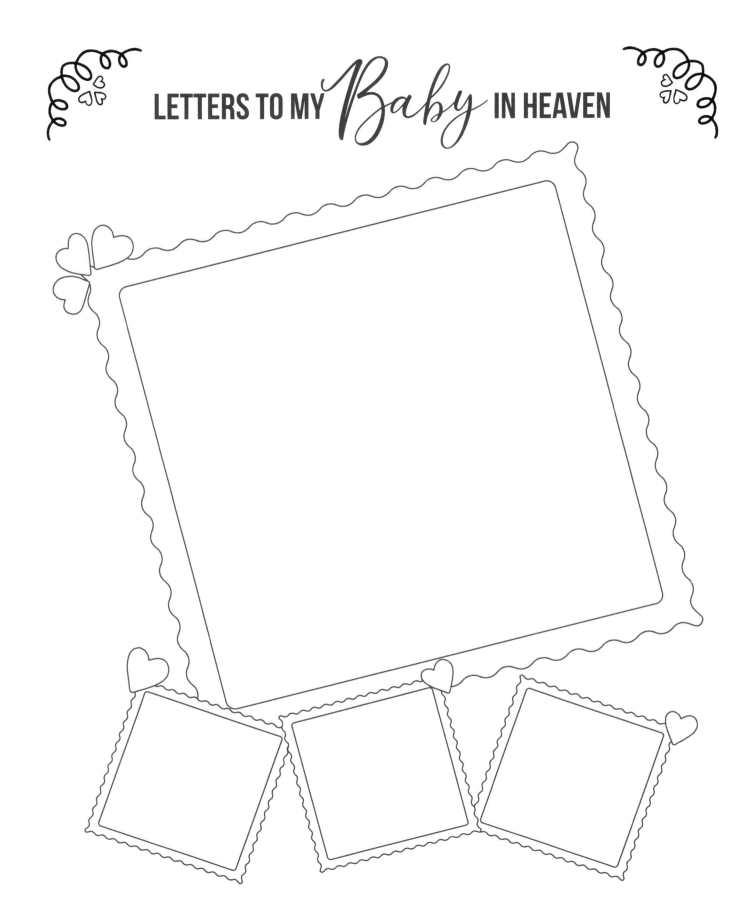